ESSENTIALS OF HAND SURGERY

Essam Abdelhakim

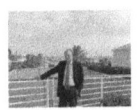

Copyright © 2024 Essam abdelhakim

All rights reserved

The characters and events portrayed in this book are fictitious. Any similarity to real persons, living or dead, is coincidental and not intended by the author.

No part of this book may be reproduced, or stored in a retrieval system, or transmitted in any form or by any means, electronic, mechanical, photocopying, recording, or otherwise, without express written permission of the publisher.

Cover design by: Art Painter
Library of Congress Control Number: 2018675309
Printed in the United States of America

CONTENTS

Title Page
Copyright
Introduction 1
Chapter 1: Anatomy of the Hand 2
Chapter 2: Common Hand Conditions and Injuries 7
Chapter 3: Congenital Anomalies of the Hand 18
Chapter 4: Hand Surgery Quizzes 21
Disclosure 39
About The Author 41

INTRODUCTION

Hand surgery *is a delicate and intricate field of medicine that focuses on the treatment and repair of the hand and wrist. The hand is an incredibly complex structure, consisting of 27 bones, 27 joints, and a network of muscles, tendons, ligaments, nerves, and blood vessels. Due to the hand's crucial role in our daily lives, any injury or condition affecting the hand can have a significant impact on an individual's functionality and quality of life.*

Hand surgery *aims to restore function, improve mobility, and alleviate pain in patients with hand-related issues. This eBook will provide an in-depth overview of hand surgery, including the most common procedures, the latest advancements in the field, and the road to recovery post-surgery.*

CHAPTER 1: ANATOMY OF THE HAND

Bones And Joints

The hand is comprised of 27 bones, divided into three groups: the carpals, metacarpals, and phalanges.

The carpals form the wrist, consisting of eight small bones arranged in two rows, which provide stability and mobility to the wrist joint.

The scaphoid bone, located in the proximal row, is particularly important as it transmits force from the arm to the hand during powerful grips.

The metacarpals, five long bones, form the palm of the hand and connect the carpals to the phalanges, the bones of the fingers.

Each finger, excluding the thumb, has three phalanges: proximal, middle, and distal phalanx. The thumb has only two phalanges, a proximal and distal phalanx, contributing to its increased range of motion and opposition, which is crucial for tasks requiring precision grip.

The joints of the hand include the wrist joint, or radiocarpal joint, which allows for flexion, extension, adduction, and abduction of the hand.

The midcarpal joint, formed by the proximal carpals, enables some rotational movements. The metacarpophalangeal (MCP) joints are the large knuckles at the base of the fingers, providing a wide range of motions, including flexion, extension, abduction, and adduction.

The proximal interphalangeal (PIP) joints and distal interphalangeal (DIP) joints are the smaller knuckles that contribute to finger flexion and extension.

Muscles And Tendons

The hand is moved by a combination of extrinsic and intrinsic muscles.

The extrinsic muscles originate in the forearm and include flexors and extensors.

The flexor muscles, located on the underside of the forearm, work to curl the fingers and bring objects towards the palm.

The flexor digitorum profundus and flexor digitorum

superficialis are the primary flexors responsible for finger flexion. The flexor pollicis longus and brevis control the movement of the thumb.

In contrast, the extensor muscles, located on the back of the forearm, work to straighten the fingers and thumb. The extensor digitorum controls the extension of the fingers, while the extensor digiti minimi extends the little finger.

The extensor pollicis longus and brevis are responsible for extending and abducting the thumb, respectively. These muscles are crucial for tasks requiring finger dexterity and the ability to form a fist.

Intrinsic muscles, located within the hand itself, contribute to fine motor movements and grip strength.

The thenar muscles, located at the base of the thumb, allow for opposition and abduction of the thumb, movements essential for pinching and grasping.

The hypothenar muscles, found at the base of the little finger, assist in abducting and extending the finger.

The lumbrical muscles, small worm-like muscles, originate from the flexor tendons and insert on the palmar aspect of the phalanges, aiding in finger flexion and extension.

Tendons are fibrous cords that attach muscles to bones, transmitting the force generated by the muscles to create movement.

In the hand, tendons play a critical role in finger flexion and extension. The flexor tendons, located on the palm side, are responsible for bending the fingers and thumb.

The flexor tendon sheath, a tunnel-like structure, surrounds the flexor tendons, providing lubrication and protection. Extensor tendons, located on the back of the hand and fingers, enable finger extension and are similarly protected by tendon sheaths.

Nerves And Blood Vessels

The hand is supplied by several major nerves, including the median, ulnar, and radial nerves, all of which originate from the brachial plexus in the arm.

The median nerve runs through the carpal tunnel, a narrow passageway on the palm side of the wrist, and provides sensation to the thumb, index finger, middle finger, and half of the ring finger. It also controls the muscles at the base of the thumb, allowing for opposition and fine motor skills.

Carpal tunnel syndrome occurs when this nerve becomes compressed within the carpal tunnel, leading to pain, numbness, and tingling in the affected fingers.

The ulnar nerve travels close to the median nerve but continues down the arm and into the hand, supplying sensation to the *little finger and half of the ring finger. It also innervates some of the intrinsic hand muscles.*

The radial nerve, as the name suggests, runs close to the radius bone and provides motor and sensory functions to the back of the hand and wrist.

Blood supply to the hand is provided by the radial artery, which originates from the brachial artery in the arm, and the ulnar artery, a branch of the brachial artery that travels alongside the ulnar nerve.

These arteries form an arch, known as the palmar arch, on the palm side of the hand, from which smaller arteries arise to supply oxygenated blood to the tissues of the hand and fingers.

The venous system follows a similar pattern, with veins accompanying the arteries to return deoxygenated blood back to the heart.

CHAPTER 2: COMMON HAND CONDITIONS AND INJURIES

Carpal Tunnel Syndrome (Cts)

Carpal tunnel syndrome is a common condition that arises from compression of the median nerve as it passes through the carpal tunnel at the wrist.

Symptoms typically include numbness, tingling, and pain in the affected fingers, particularly at night, and may extend up the forearm.

CTS is often associated with repetitive wrist movements, such as continuous typing or assembly line work, and is more prevalent in women than men.

Non-surgical management of CTS involves resting the affected hand and wrist, wearing a wrist splint to immobilize the wrist in a neutral position, particularly during sleep, and taking non-steroidal anti-inflammatory drugs (NSAIDs) to reduce pain and swelling.

Steroid injections *into the carpal tunnel can also be effective in reducing inflammation and providing temporary relief.*

Trigger Finger

Trigger finger, or stenosing tenosynovitis, is a condition where one or more fingers become locked in a bent position, often with a snapping sensation when trying to straighten the finger.

It occurs when the flexor tendon becomes inflamed and nodules form, causing the tendon to catch as it glides through the tendon sheath.

Trigger finger is commonly seen in individuals with diabetes or rheumatoid arthritis and those who engage in repetitive gripping activities.

Treatment for trigger finger initially involves conservative measures such as rest, splinting the affected finger in extension, and NSAIDs to reduce inflammation.

Steroid injections into the tendon sheath can be highly effective in reducing symptoms.

In cases where conservative treatments fail, a minor surgical procedure, called a trigger finger release, can be performed to open the constricted portion of the tendon sheath, allowing the tendon to move freely again.

Ganglion Cysts

Ganglion cysts are fluid-filled sacs that typically develop along the tendons or joint capsules of the hand and wrist.

They can vary in size and may be painless or cause discomfort, depending on their location and size.

Ganglion cysts are commonly found at the wrist, the base of the fingers, or the tip of the finger, where they may interfere with joint movement or cause nerve compression.

Initial treatment for ganglion cysts is often conservative, involving aspiration of the cyst with a needle and syringe to remove the fluid, followed by compression bandaging to prevent refilling.

Corticosteroid injections can also be used to shrink the cyst. If these measures are unsuccessful or the cyst recurs, surgical excision may be recommended.

Surgery involves removing the cyst and a small portion of the surrounding joint capsule or tendon sheath to prevent recurrence.

Hand Fractures

Fractures of the hand are common injuries, often resulting from falls, sports injuries, or direct trauma.

The metacarpals and phalanges are the most frequently fractured bones in the hand.

Symptoms include pain, swelling, bruising, and deformity, with potential loss of function and mobility. Some fractures may involve the joint surfaces, which can lead to long-term complications if not treated appropriately.

Non-surgical management of hand fractures involves immobilization with a cast or splint to allow the bones to heal in proper alignment.

Ice, elevation, and NSAIDs can help manage pain and swelling. However, surgical intervention is often required for more complex fractures, especially those involving joint surfaces or multiple bone fragments.

Open reduction and internal fixation (ORIF) are a common procedure where the fracture fragments are realigned and held in place with screws, plates, or wires, ensuring proper healing and restoring function.

Dislocations

Dislocations of the hand joints, particularly the MCP and PIP joints, are common injuries, often resulting from sports activities, falls, or direct impact.

A dislocation occurs when the ends of the bones are forced out of their normal alignment within a joint.

Symptoms include intense pain, swelling, and deformity, with the affected joint appearing out of place.

Immediate reduction of a dislocation is crucial to prevent further damage to the surrounding ligaments, blood vessels, and nerves.

This involves manipulating the joint to return the bones to their correct positions.

Following successful reduction, the joint is typically immobilized in a cast or splint for several weeks to allow the surrounding structures to heal. In some cases, surgical intervention may be necessary to repair damaged ligaments or reconstruct severely torn structures.

Tendon Injuries

Tendon injuries in the hand can range from inflammation to partial or complete tears.

Tendinitis, or tendon inflammation, is often caused by repetitive motions and can affect the flexor or extensor tendons.

Symptoms include pain, swelling, and tenderness along the affected tendon.

Tendinitis is typically managed with rest, splinting, and NSAIDs to reduce inflammation. Steroid injections may also be used to alleviate symptoms.

In more severe cases, tendons can tear, either partially or completely.

This often occurs with forceful, sudden movements, and patients may feel a snap or pop, followed by intense pain and difficulty moving the affected finger or thumb.

Partial tears may be managed conservatively with immobilization and physical therapy.

However, complete tears typically require surgical repair to restore function.

Tendon repair surgery involves suturing the torn tendon back together or, in severe cases, using a tendon graft to replace the damaged portion.

Hand Infections

Infections in the hand can range from mild to severe and are typically caused by bacteria, viruses, or fungi.

These organisms can enter the hand through breaks in the skin, such as cuts, abrasions, or puncture wounds, or through the spread of infection from another part of the body. Hand infections can affect the skin, soft tissues, tendons, and bones, and they require prompt attention to prevent complications.

Infections in the hand can arise from various pathogens, including bacteria, viruses, and fungi.

These organisms exploit breaks in the skin, such as cuts, abrasions, or puncture wounds, to invade the hand, or they may spread from another infected site in the body.

Hand infections can involve the skin, soft tissues, tendons, and even bones, underscoring the importance of prompt recognition and treatment to prevent complications.

Cellulitis

Cellulitis is a common bacterial infection of the skin and underlying soft tissues.

It often occurs following a break in the skin, such as a cut, insect bite, or scratch.

The affected area becomes red, swollen, warm, and painful. Cellulitis can spread rapidly and, in some cases, lead to a serious complication called sepsis if left untreated.

Treatment for cellulitis typically involves oral antibiotics to eradicate the infection. Incision and drainage may be necessary if an abscess is present.

Paronychia

Paronychia is an infection that occurs around the nail fold, usually caused by bacteria or fungi.

It often affects individuals who frequently immerse their hands in water or have their hands in moist environments.

The affected finger becomes swollen, tender, and red, and there may be pus accumulation.

Acute paronychia is typically treated with warm water soaks and antibiotics. In chronic cases, surgical drainage and nail fold repair may be necessary.

Felon

A felon is a painful infection that occurs in the distal pulp space of the fingertip, usually caused by bacteria.

It often results from a puncture wound or deep abrasion to the fingertip. Symptoms include intense pain, swelling, and a white or yellow collection of pus visible through the nail bed.

Treatment involves incision and drainage to relieve pressure and oral antibiotics to clear the infection.

Herpetic Whitlow

Herpetic whitlow is a viral infection caused by the herpes simplex virus (HSV).

It typically affects individuals who handle objects contaminated with the virus, such as healthcare workers or dentists.

The infection causes painful, fluid-filled blisters on the fingers or thumb, which can rupture and form crusts.

Treatment includes antiviral medications, pain management, and, in severe cases, incision and drainage.

Septic Arthritis

Septic arthritis of the hand is a serious infection that involves the joint space.

It is often caused by bacteria, such as Staphylococcus aureus, which can enter the joint through a penetrating injury or spread hematogenously.

Symptoms include intense joint pain, swelling, warmth, and limited range of motion.

Treatment requires prompt surgical drainage of the joint, followed by a course of intravenous antibiotics.

Osteomyelitis

Osteomyelitis is a bacterial infection of the bone, which can affect the hand bones.

It typically occurs following an open fracture or as a result of hematogenous spread from another site of infection.

Symptoms include severe pain, swelling, redness, and fever. Treatment involves a prolonged course of intravenous antibiotics and surgical debridement of the affected bone to remove infected tissue and promote healing.

CHAPTER 3: CONGENITAL ANOMALIES OF THE HAND

Syndactyly

Syndactyly is a congenital condition characterized by the fusion of two or more fingers or toes, resulting from the failure of digital rays to separate during embryonic development.

It can involve soft tissue webbing or the fusion of bones. Surgical correction, typically performed during early childhood, involves separating the digits and reconstructing the associated soft tissues to improve hand function and appearance.

Polydactyly

Polydactyly is the presence of extra fingers or toes, representing an overgrowth of digital rays during embryogenesis.

The additional digits may be fully formed or consist of small, underdeveloped bones. Surgical treatment, often performed during the first year of life, involves the removal of the extra digit and associated soft tissues, followed by reconstruction to achieve a functional and aesthetically pleasing outcome.

Camptodactyly

Camptodactyly is a condition characterized by fixed flexion contractures of one or more fingers, resulting from an abnormality in the flexor tendons or their attachments.

The affected finger(s) remain bent in a flexed position, impacting hand function and grip strength.

Treatment may involve serial casting to gradually extend the finger, or surgery to release and lengthen the affected tendons, followed by occupational therapy for optimal recovery.

Clinodactyly

Clinodactyly is a lateral or medial deviation of the finger, most commonly affecting the fifth finger, causing it to angle towards the ring finger.

This anomaly is often associated with other genetic syndromes, such as Down syndrome. Mild cases may not require treatment, while more severe deviations can be corrected surgically during childhood to improve hand function and aesthetics.

Symbrachydactyly

Symbrachydactyly is a rare congenital anomaly characterized by the underdevelopment or absence of digits, typically affecting the hand and forearm.

It can involve hypoplasia or aplasia of bones, muscles, tendons, and nerves, resulting in a shortened and deformed limb.

Treatment options include surgical reconstruction to improve function and symmetry, as well as prosthetic devices to enhance the individual's capabilities.

CHAPTER 4: HAND SURGERY QUIZZES

A 35-Year-Old Patient Presents With A Swollen, Tender Lump On Their Wrist, Suspected To Be A Ganglion Cyst.

Which Of The Following Structures Is The Cyst Most Likely Attached To?

A) Tendon sheath

B) Bone

C) Ligament

D) Nerve

E) Blood vessel

Answer: A) Tendon sheath

Explanation: Ganglion cysts are fluid-filled sacs that typically arise as outpocketings from tendon sheaths or joint capsules. The wrist is one of the most common locations for ganglion cysts, and they are often attached to the tendon sheath, making option A the correct choice.

Which Nerve Is Most Commonly Associated With Carpal Tunnel Syndrome, And What Symptoms Might A Patient Experience?

A) Ulnar nerve, pain in the little finger

B) Radial nerve, weakness in the wrist

C) Median nerve, numbness and tingling in the thumb, index, middle finger

D) Axillary nerve, shoulder pain

E) Sciatic nerve, leg pain

Answer: C) Median nerve, numbness and tingling in the thumb, index, middle finger

Explanation: Carpal tunnel syndrome occurs when the median nerve, which runs through the carpal tunnel in the wrist, becomes compressed. This compression leads to symptoms of numbness, tingling, and pain in the areas innervated by the median nerve, including the thumb, index finger, middle finger, and half of the ring finger. Therefore, option C is the correct answer.

A Patient Sustains A Deep Laceration To Their Hand, Damaging The Flexor Tendons.

Which Surgical Technique Is Commonly Used To Repair This Type Of Injury?

A) Endoscopic surgery

B) Open reduction and internal fixation (ORIF)

C) Microsurgery

D) Tendon transfer

E) Amputation

Answer: C) Microsurgery

Explanation: Microsurgery is the appropriate technique for repairing damaged flexor tendons in the hand. This specialized surgery uses microscopes and fine instruments to meticulously suture the torn tendon ends together, ensuring precise alignment and optimal healing. Option C is, therefore, the correct choice.

A 55-Year-Old Patient With Rheumatoid Arthritis Experiences Trigger Finger In Their Dominant Hand.

Which Of The Following Treatments Is Most Suitable As The Initial Approach?

A) Rest and NSAIDs

B) Corticosteroid injections

C) Surgical release

D) Occupational therapy

E) Tendon lengthening

Answer: B) Corticosteroid injections

Explanation: The initial treatment for trigger finger, especially in patients with underlying conditions like rheumatoid arthritis, typically involves corticosteroid injections into the tendon sheath. This helps reduce inflammation and can provide significant relief. Rest and NSAIDs (option A) may be recommended as part of conservative management, but they are not the primary treatment in this scenario. Therefore, option B is the correct answer.

Which Hand Fracture Is Commonly Known As A "Boxer's Fracture"?

A) Fracture of the hamate bone

B) Fracture of the metacarpal neck

C) Bennett's fracture

D) Rolando's fracture

E) Colles' fracture

Answer: B) Fracture of the metacarpal neck

Explanation: A "boxer's fracture" specifically refers to a fracture of the neck of one of the metacarpal bones, usually the fourth or fifth metacarpal, which can occur when a person punches a hard object and impacts the knuckles. This injury is common in boxers, hence the name. Option B is, therefore, the correct choice.

During Hand Surgery, Which Type Of Anaesthesia Is Commonly Used To Provide Adequate Pain Control While Allowing The Patient To Move Their Fingers?

A) General anaesthesia

B) Local anaesthesia with sedation

C) Regional anaesthesia (block)

D) Epidural anaesthesia

E) Conscious sedation

Answer: C) Regional anaesthesia (block)

Explanation: Regional anaesthesia, or a nerve block, is often used for hand surgery as it provides effective pain control by blocking the nerves supplying the surgical site. This allows the patient to be awake and able to move their fingers during surgery, which is beneficial for assessing nerve and tendon function. Option C is, therefore, the correct answer.

A Patient Undergoes Surgery For A Severe Mallet Finger Injury.

Which Of The Following Best Describes The Procedure?

A) Extensor tendon repair

B) Flexor tendon grafting

C) Joint fusion

D) Tendon release

E) Pinning and splinting

Answer: E) Pinning and splinting

Explanation: A mallet finger injury involves a rupture or avulsion of the extensor tendon from the distal phalanx, causing the fingertip to droop. Treatment typically involves pinning the fractured bone fragment in an extended position, followed by splinting for several weeks to promote healing. Option E is, therefore, the correct choice.

Which Hand Condition Is Characterized By A Painless, Firm, Mobile Lump, Often Found At The Wrist Or Base Of The Finger?

A) Ganglion cyst

B) Lipoma

C) Giant cell tumour

D) Neuroma

E) Haemangioma

Answer: A) Ganglion cyst

Explanation: Ganglion cysts are fluid-filled sacs that commonly present as painless, mobile lumps at the wrist or base of the finger. They are typically firm and may vary in size. Ganglion cysts are benign and often asymptomatic, making option A the correct choice.

A Patient With A Severe Case Of Dupuytren's Contracture Undergoes Surgery.

Which Layer Of Tissue Is Divided During The Procedure?

A) Fascia

B) Skin

C) Muscle

D) Tendon

E) Bone

Answer: A) Fascia

Explanation: Dupuytren's contracture is a condition that causes thickening and contraction of the palmar fascia, resulting in the fingers being pulled into a flexed position. Surgery involves dividing and releasing the affected fascia to restore finger extension. Option A is, therefore, the correct answer.

Which hand surgery technique utilizes a small camera, and specialized instruments inserted through tiny incisions?

A) Endoscopic surgery

B) Microsurgery

C) Open surgery

D) Percutaneous surgery

E) Laser surgery

Answer: A) Endoscopic surgery

Explanation: Endoscopic surgery employs a small, thin tube with a camera (endoscope) and specialized instruments inserted through small incisions in the skin.

This technique allows for minimally invasive procedures, reducing trauma to surrounding tissues and offering faster recovery times. Option A is, therefore, the correct choice.

A Patient With A History Of Repetitive Motion Presents With Pain, Swelling, And A Clicking Sensation In Their Thumb.

Which Of The Following Structures Is Most Likely Affected?

A) Flexor pollicis longus tendon

B) Extensor pollicis brevis tendon

C) Abductor pollicis longus tendon

D) Ulnar collateral ligament

E) Radial collateral ligament

Answer: D) Ulnar collateral ligament

Explanation: The described symptoms are indicative of "skier's thumb" or a sprain/tear of the ulnar collateral ligament of the thumb. This ligament provides stability to the metacarpophalangeal joint of the thumb during grasping and pinching movements. Option D is, therefore, the correct answer.

Which Hand Surgery Procedure Involves Removing A Portion Of The Affected Bone To Realign And Stabilize A Fracture?

A) Bone grafting

B) Osteotomy

C) Arthroplasty

D) Arthrodesis

E) Bone pinning

Answer: B) Osteotomy

Explanation: An osteotomy involves cutting and removing a small portion of bone to realign and correct a deformity or misalignment. This procedure is often performed to treat certain types of fractures or to improve hand function in conditions like osteoarthritis. Option B is, therefore, the correct choice.

A Patient With A Severe Case Of Rheumatoid Arthritis Experiences A Boutonniere Deformity In Their Finger.

Which Of The Following Best Describes This Condition?

A) Hyperextension of the proximal interphalangeal joint and flexion of the distal interphalangeal joint

B) Flexion contracture of the proximal interphalangeal joint and hyperextension of the distal interphalangeal joint

C) Flexion contracture of both the proximal and distal interphalangeal joints

D) Extension contracture of both the proximal and distal interphalangeal joints

E) Swelling and stiffness of the entire finger

Answer: B) Flexion contracture of the proximal interphalangeal joint and hyperextension of the distal interphalangeal joint

Explanation: A boutonniere deformity is characterized by a flexion contracture of the proximal interphalangeal (PIP) joint and hyperextension of the distal interphalangeal (DIP) joint, giving the affected finger a characteristic "buttonhole" appearance. This deformity is commonly associated with rheumatoid arthritis and is correctly described in option B.

Which Hand Surgery Technique Is Used To Treat Severe, Debilitating Arthritis Of The

Basal Joint Of The Thumb?

A) Arthrodesis

B) Arthroplasty

C) Tendon transfer

D) Joint aspiration and injection

E) Amputation

Answer: B) Arthroplasty

Explanation: Arthroplasty, or joint replacement surgery, is the preferred treatment for severe arthritis of the basal joint of the thumb. This procedure involves removing the damaged articular surfaces and replacing them with a prosthetic implant to restore pain-free movement. Option B is, therefore, the correct answer.

A Patient With A History Of Hand Trauma Complains Of Cold And Discoloured Fingers.

Which Of The Following Conditions Are They Most Likely Experiencing?

A) Raynaud's phenomenon

B) Complex regional pain syndrome

C) Peripheral neuropathy

D) Carpal tunnel syndrome

E) Tenosynovitis

Answer: A) Raynaud's phenomenon

Explanation: The described symptoms of cold and discoloured fingers, especially in the context of hand trauma, are indicative of Raynaud's phenomenon. This condition involves spasms of the blood vessels in response to cold temperatures or emotional stress, leading to reduced blood flow to the fingers. Option A is, therefore, the correct choice.

Which Hand Surgery Procedure Involves Transferring A Tendon From One Site To Another To Restore Function?

A) Tendon lengthening

B) Tendon transfer

C) Tendon repair

D) Tendon grafting

E) Tendon release

Answer: B) Tendon transfer

Explanation: Tendon transfer surgery is performed to restore function in cases where a particular tendon is damaged or paralyzed. A working tendon from a less critical muscle is transferred to replace the function of the affected tendon, improving hand function and grip strength. Option B is, therefore, the correct answer.

A Patient With A Severe Case Of Carpal Tunnel Syndrome Undergoes Surgery.

Which Structure Is Divided During The Procedure To Relieve Pressure On The Median Nerve?

A) Transverse carpal ligament

B) Flexor retinaculum

C) Palmar aponeurosis

D) Dorsal wrist capsule

E) Extensor retinaculum

Answer: A) Transverse carpal ligament

Explanation: Carpal tunnel release surgery involves dividing the transverse carpal ligament, which forms the roof of the carpal tunnel, to relieve pressure on the median nerve. This procedure increases the space within the tunnel, alleviating symptoms of carpal tunnel syndrome. Option A is, therefore, the correct choice.

Which Hand Surgery Technique Is Commonly Used To Treat Severe, Non-Healing Fractures Or Infections?

A) Bone lengthening

B) Bone grafting

C) External fixation

D) Internal fixation

E) Amputation

Answer: B) Bone grafting

Explanation: Bone grafting is a surgical technique used to treat complex or non-healing fractures, as well as severe bone infections. It involves transplanting bone tissue, either from another site in the patient's body (autograft) or from a donor (allograft), to promote healing and restore bone structure. Option B is, therefore, the correct answer.

A Patient With A History Of Hand Trauma Complains Of Chronic Pain And Sensitivity In Their Hand. They Exhibit Signs Of Allodynia

And Hyperalgesia.

Which Of The Following Conditions Are They Most Likely Experiencing?

A) Complex regional pain syndrome (CRPS)

B) Phantom limb syndrome

C) Peripheral neuropathy

D) Carpal tunnel syndrome

E) Tenosynovitis

Answer: A) Complex regional pain syndrome (CRPS)

Explanation: The described symptoms of chronic pain, allodynia (pain from stimuli that should not cause pain), and hyperalgesia (increased sensitivity to painful stimuli) are hallmark features of complex regional pain syndrome (CRPS). This condition can develop following hand trauma and is characterized by prolonged, disproportionate pain and sensory abnormalities. Option A is, therefore, the correct choice.

A Patient With A Severe Case Of Dupuytren's Contracture Undergoes Surgery, And The Surgeon Performs A Fasciectomy.

Which Of The Following Best Describes This Procedure?

A) Removal of the palmar fascia

B) Release of the flexor tendons

C) Excision of a ganglion cyst

D) Bone shortening osteotomy

E) Joint replacement

Answer: A) Removal of the palmar fascia

Explanation: A fasciectomy involves the surgical removal of the affected palmar fascia, which is the underlying cause of Dupuytren's contracture. This procedure releases the contracture, improving finger extension and hand function. Option A is, therefore, the correct choice.

DISCLOSURE

Disclosure
This book has been created with the assistance of ***Artificial Intelligence (AI) tools*** and thoroughly reviewed and edited by the author to ensure clarity, relevance, and educational value.

While every effort has been made to provide accurate and up-to-date information, this content is intended solely for educational and informational purposes.

The author is a medical professional; however, the information provided in this book *is not a substitute for professional medical advice, diagnosis, or treatment.*

Readers are strongly advised to consult licensed healthcare providers or specialists for any medical concerns or conditions.

By using this book, **you acknowledge and agree** that the author shall not be held responsible or liable for any loss, damage, or harm whether physical, emotional, financial, or otherwise that may occur *as a result of the use or misuse of the information presented herein.*

ABOUT THE AUTHOR

Dr Essam Abdelhakim

Senior Consultant and Expert In Medical Education

www.ingramcontent.com/pod-product-compliance
Lightning Source LLC
Chambersburg PA
CBHW070950220526
45471CB00007B/2973